IMPROVING THE COORDINATION OF CARE AN EDUCATIONAL PROGRAM

By

Irwin Rubin

Ronald Fry

Mark Plovnick

Norman Stearns

KALPAZ

ISBN: 978-93-5128-687-5(HB)

First Published, 1975

Published by

Kalpaz Publications
C-30, Satyawati Nagar,
Delhi – 110052
E-mail: kalpaz@hotmail.com
Ph.: 9212142040

Printed at: G. Print Process, Delhi

IMPROVING THE COORDINATION OF CARE: AN EDUCATIONAL PROGRAM

by

RUBIN, Irwin Ph.D. Organization Behavior, Lecturer Massachusetts Institute of Technology Alfred P. Sloan School of Management 50 Memorial Drive Cambridge, Massachusetts 02139

FRY, Ronald Ph.D. Candidate in Organization Behavior Massachusetts Institute of Technology Alfred P. Sloan School of Management 50 Memorial Drive Cambridge, Massachusetts 02139

PLOVNICK, Mark Ph.D. Organization Behavior, Research Associate Massachusetts Institute of Technology Alfred P. Sloan School of Management 50 Memorial Drive Cambridge, Massachusetts 02139

STEARNS, Norman M.D. , Associate Dean for Continuing Education Tufts University School of Medicine 136 Harrison Avenue Boston, Massachusetts 02111 also Visiting Associate Professor, M.I.T. Sloan School of Management

SYNOPSIS ABSTRACT

The effective delivery of health care requires coordinated interdisciplinary team efforts involving doctors, nurses, and many other health workers. Conscious and systematic efforts must be undertaken to deal with the problems inherent in trying to accomplish a task requiring coordination of interdependent functions. A self-instructional educational program, based on applied behavioral science con- cepts and techniques already proven to be effective in non-health care settings, has been specifically designed to help health workers improve the coordination of care delivery.

The impact of this team development program was studied in thirteen health care settings. Improvements were noted in many areas: (a) less confusion and conflict over goals and priorities; (b) better utilization and allocation of team members' resources; and (c) more efficient and effective work procedures (e.g. meetings, decision procedures). While rigorous empirical data about patient care is not available, there was substantial perceptual evidence — from both deliverers and administrators — that the delivery of care was improved.

These results support the belief that "developed" teams are more efficient and effective deliverers of care than non-developed teams.

INTRODUCTION

Health practitioners in many settings are increasingly recognizing the need for improved coordination between various health workers. Many physicians in particular, whether in hospitals, primary care clinics, community health centers, group practices or solo practices, are realizing that to improve the delivery of care, more effective "teamwork" is required. 1-4 A significant number of papers on issues in "team care" were presented at the recent A.M. A. 70th Annual Congress on Medical Education.

The purpose of this article is to outline an approach to effective team func- tioning and describe the main elements and field-test results of a specific educa- tional program developed to improve teamwork among health practitioners. -> The underlying concepts in the approach to be described have been developed and success- fully applied by behavioral scientists working in industrial settings over the past two decades. ~" The application and relevance of these same concepts and approaches to health care systems is, however, just beginning to be examined. 10-1 3

General Approach to Teams

If a task or job to be done requires the interdependent efforts of two or more people, then a team situation exists. Interdependent means that the individuals involved must work together and coordinate their activities with each other : the job cannot be done as well by one person alone. In many health care delivery situations, different individuals with different knowledge, skills, attitudes, backgrounds, and training must function interdependently to get the task done. There is a dilemma, however, in that the individual differences which are essential to effectively accomplish team tasks also represent potential obstacles to efficient teamwork.

Within the framework of the general definition offered above, all health prac- titioners are, in some sense, members of "teams," be it the solo practitioner and his secretary, or the several doctors, nurses, and technicians who constitute an operating room (OR) team. Factors which can hinder team performance in any setting will be considered first. Subsequently, the extent to which "teams" in various settings are affected by and need to concern themselves with these problem factors will be specifically addressed.

Problems Caused by Interdependence - The Symptoms of Poor Teamwork

The symptoms of poor teamwork are reflected in the following kinds of concerns expressed by team members and administrators in team settings ;14,15 unnecessary duplication of effort; incomplete or forgotten tasks; team members pulling in dif- ferent directions; team decisions not being followed up; grumbling behind the scenes;- team meetings are less than satisfactory; sloppy verbal communication, and incomplete charts.

These symptoms are an indication that a team has not successfully dealt with the problems inherent in trying to accomplish a task requiring coordination of interdependent functions. The problems caused by interdependence fall into four general areas: (1) problems caused by different goals (short and long range) and priorities. . ."What are we supposed to be doing?"; (2) the issue of role responsi- bilities and the problems caused by different specialists trying to work in an integrated way... "Who is doing what?"; (3) problems caused by the need to develop effective and efficient procedures for group decision-making, problem-solving, and communication. .. "How do we accomplish our work?"; (4) interpersonal issues which arise when people function interdependently, such as trust and need for support. . ."How does it feel to work around here?".

Problems with Goals

Meeting patients' health care needs is often a frustrating task. Success can be hard to define and to measure. In the absence of specific short-range measurable goals, team members only occasionally get the sense of having acomplished anything. In addition, without an agreed-upon mission or set of objectives, individual team members are very likely to go off in a variety of different directions, each doing "his own thing. "16-18 Conflicts then develop around how time should be spent, by whom, and around which kinds of tasks. Unresolved conflicts in goals and priorities can result in much wasted time and energy.

Problems of Roles

The full utilization of a team's human resources is often stymied because of ambiguity or unresolved conflicts over "Who should be doing what?"!' Standardized job descriptions and a priori assumptions about professional role responsibilities and relationships often do not and cannot be expected to cover all of the day-to-day contingencies which characterize an interdependent task like health care. Unre- solved role conflicts and ambiguous responsibilities can act to drain considerable energy from team members.

Problems with Procedures

There are a variety of ways by which a team can organize its work and proce- dures. How a particular group makes decisions, how it conducts its meetings, how it decides who is to initiate, consult, or support various activities depends upon the particular task and particular individual roles in a given situation. 20,21 A team must therefore spend time in meetings talking and deciding upon how to coor- dinate the individual efforts of individual members. The time and energy spent in such meetings is often wasted because health workers are usually trained as in- dividual practitioners and are seldom trained to manage collective problem-solving or decision-making sessions. As a result, meetings are often characterized by unclear decisions, mixed commitments to follow-up, and low energy to volunteer or participate inuture team meetings.

Problems with Interpersonal Relationships

Interpersonal tensions and conflicts often develop and operate negatively to drain energy from team members. Human behavioral experience suggests that the frustrating nature of certain tasks creates strong needs for peer support and posi- tive feedback on one's competence from superiors and co-workers. 22-24 xhus, be- haviors that lead to or detract from trust, self-confidence, support, and pleasant working relationships, are issues which must be worked on by the team as a whole.

When not due to problems related to goals, roles, or work structure, manifest interpersonal problems may indicate that one or more team members are actually mismatched with the job. This alternative should be considered only after the other three categories of problems have been addressed.

The Need for Team Development

Team development activities are aimed at helping a team to minimize time and energy lost mismanaging problems stemming from interdependence, and maximize the energy devoted to accomplishing team tasks. In different teams, the need for and nature of team development exercises will vary according to the characteristics of the task to be done.

As a case in point, let us examine two different examples, an O.R. team setting and a comprehensive community health care team. The task of an O.R. team is rela- tively specific and clearly definable. While the ultimate surgical problem may be uncertain, the team's goals, roles, and procedures are all very certain and few conflicts in priority exist. The role responsibilities of individual team members are specifiable and any person trained in the specific role (e.g. first assistant surgeon, scrub nurse, or anesthesiologist) can fulfill the needed functions. The organizational and decision-making structure of an O.R. team, consequently, is predetermined and the system is able to operate at high levels of efficiency ex- hibiting few of the general symptoms of poor teamwork.

The situation in a comprehensive community health care setting is dramatically different. The team's goal or task is very uncertain — differences in individual interpretation and conflicts in priorities are therefore to be expected. It is unlikely, given the complexities of the task, that complete job descriptions will ever be feasible in such settings. Work structures and procedures must be worked out by the team members which are consistent with team goals and individual role responsibilities .

The rationale for investing in team development efforts is the expectation that by explicitly dealing with predictable team problems — caused by the nature of certain tasks — the team will avoid greater time and energy losses resulting from ineffective operations later. Left to their own devices over time, teams do not typically resolve these problems and consequently continue to perform at low levels of efficiency. In an exploratory questionnaire survey, conducted by the authors, of 35 teams which had functioned for varying periods of time, over 60 per cent reported that they were functioning only "fairly well." (The mid-point of a seven-point scale ranging from 1 = teams are having difficulty working to7 = teams are working very well.) The overwhelming majority (91%) expressed a need for inputs which would help them improve, while only one reported that their team was working well and did not need any improvement. Team development, therefore, must be viewed as a planned maintenance activity aimed at preventing major problems from occurring .

The following sections of this paper describe the central elements of one program in team development designed specifically for health care delivery teams.

A Program for Health Team Development

Overall Objectives

The Health Team Development (HTD) program has two overriding objectives:

(1) to help a team solve specific task-related problems (e.g. goal setting, role allocation, etc.) and therefore begin to function more effectively right away; and (2) to provide the team with a set of skills

and concepts (e.g. conflict resolu- tion, decision-making, role clarification) which they can apply in the future as similar problems develop. While these two goals have some costs, (primarily the amount of time investment required) , it is important that both goals be maintained if teams are to derive long-run benefit from the effort.

Task-Oriented Focus

The activities in this program are real in the sense that they involve all team members directly. The focus is on helping the team to solve its own problems which result from the nature of the job to be done. This program does not follow a traditional lecture or classroom training format. The outputs from each session include procedures, agreements, and solutions directly related to day-to-day work activities.

Self-Instructional Approach

The program is designed so that it can be run by the team itself, with no outside consultants, trainers, or observers. The authors' early experiences with health care teams were as traditional outside consultants working directly and personally with teams in team development activities. 25 The success of those ex- periences plus the belief that (a) more health teams existed than could be handled by the available number of consultants, and (b) many health teams did not have the resources to hire outsiders, led to the creation of this instrumented program.

Content and Flow of the Program

The program consists of two phases — Core Work and Optional Resource Modules.

1. Phase One: Core Work

This phase consists of seven, three-hour sessions or modules which focus on the most essential elements of team effectiveness (i.e. goals, roles, procedures). Each core module helps the team collect information from its members (data collec- tion) about a particular obstacle to team effectiveness (e.g. lack of clarity of goals) . The team asks itself "Where are we on this issue?" These data are then summarized and shared (feedback and analysis). At this stage, the team answers, for itself, the question: "Are we where we need to be?" Discrepancies between where they are and where they need to be become the stimulus for new action plans. These action plans are then implemented. Evaluation (new data collection) is scheduled for some later point. The process follows a model called the "action- research" approach to team development. 2 ^ Each module requires individual prepara- tion (usually 15-30 minutes). The seven core modules are described briefly.

MODULE ONE : "How Are We Doing as a Team" - Vital Signs

In this session, individuals rate team performance on several scales and then share this information in a total group discussion. Team strengths and weaknesses are assessed and specific needs for team development are identified.

MODULE TWO : "A Team Trying to Do What" - Goal Setting

This is the first of two sessions devoted to clarifying exactly what it is that the team is supposed to do. The output of this session is an agreed-upon Core Mission or general statement of purpose developed by the team.

MODULE THREE : "A Team Trying to Do What" - Setting Priorities

The team begins to operationalize its Core Mission from Module Two. Members create specific performance goals which, if met, would satisfy them that they are accomplishing their Core Mission. In addition, the team begins to prioritize its most important goals in order to help focus the energy of its members.

MODULE FOUR : "Who Does What Around Here" - Role Negotiation

This is the first of two sessions devoted to clarifying, defining, and changing roles of team members. As preparation, each member writes "messages" to every other member stating things that the other members could do differently (or the same) to help the "message sender" get his job done more effectively. These messages are exchanged in the session. The team then learns and practices a face-to-face, give-

and-take conflict resolution skill called "role negotiation." Volunteers actually resolve conflicts initiated in their messages in front of the team as a demonstra- tion for learning purposes.

MODULE FIVE : "Who Does What Around Here" - Role Definition

In this module, team members go through all their role messages from Module Four. Individuals begin to define their roles by agreeing (in writing) to the messages that are "OK" and by setting up specific times and places to "role nego- tiate" with other team members concerning messages that are not yet "OK."

MODULE SIX : "How Things Get Done Around Here" - Decision-Making

This module helps the team look at how they make decisions and how they might do it better. A problem-solving model is presented, and the team learns to use a decision-making "checklist" whenever members are at a decision-making point. The team then practices using a tool called a "decision chart" to determine how impor- tant decisions ought to be made in the future. As a result of this module's activi- ties, the team agrees to try some new operating procedures or policies.

MODULE SEVEN : "Where Do We Go From Here" - Planning Next Steps

This session concludes the core team development program by helping the team to assess its progress to date and to identify its needs for the future in order to accomplish its Core Mission. The output of this module is a detailed action plan including role responsibilities, decision-making mechanisms, and methods or eval- uating progress. All additional sessions are directed at pursuing and measuring the team's progress in light of its performance goals.

2 . Phase Two : Optional Resource Modules

This phase consists of six optional, special interest resource modules, each directed at specific problem areas which a developed team may encounter. After completing Phase One, the team is free to choose whichever (if any) of these on which they want to work. The

Phase Two Modules can be used as either individual read- ing or guides for a team session related to a particular issue. The titles of Optional Resource Modules are as follows:

MODULE A:	"Bringing a New Member Onboard" - Joining Up
MODULE B:	"Running a Better Meeting
MODULE C:	"How We Interact When We Work Around Here" - Leadership and Membership
MODULE D:	"What Does It Feel Like to Work Around Here - Norms
MODULE E:	"Interacting With the Rest of the Organization"
MODULE F:	"How Do We Look to Our Patients"-Getting Feedback

The Investment

The core program requires a team to work together for seven, three-hour sessions, preferably once per week for seven weeks. For many, the initial reaction is: "It's too much. Can't it be done faster?"

Given the realities in most health care delivery settings, freeing up the time required is indeed a major obstacle. Nevertheless, administrators must be prepared to provide short-run support to permit a team to get in shape. To facilitate this action, the Program includes a set of Guidelines to Administrators. These guide- lines are designed to help administrators implement the steps necessary to (a) get the organization ready to support the team development program, and (b) introduce the actual program to a team or teams. In no setting in which the program has been used has this been an easy task. 27 However, results from thirteen test sites strong- ly suggest that the returns warrant the investment.

Some Initial Results

Some Specific Effects : Managing Problems Stemming from Interdependence

Evaluation data was obtained in various ways: (a) periodic questionnaires to team members; (b) analysis of session outputs (e.g.

a. there are greater conscious efforts to follow through on tough cases be- cause team members are following up with each other;
b. there are more original and creative solutions to patient health problems because of greater knowledge and use of team members' resources;
c. team members check with each other more about their objectives and respon- sibilities in specific instances resulting in a more efficient utilization of the team's resources and less wasted time and energy;
d. fewer patients are getting "lost" because team members are coordinating more of their activities and being more helpful to each other, an occurrence apparently felt and appreciated by patients.

Problems With Interpersonal Relationships: A Perspective

Many individuals who experience the symptoms of poor team work described earlier, conclude that these symptoms result from individual "personality clashes." "We just don't get along," "He rubs me the wrong way," "Our chemistry if bad," are frequently voiced comments when team members discuss obstacles to effective teamwork.

From this study and our experiences in other settings, a very different per- spective emerges. Most "personality clashes" are caused by unresolved issues con- cerning goals, roles, or procedures.TM When these issues have been resolved, inter- personal tensions and personality clashes often disappear.

With respect to the specific program being discussed, people do report feeling much more positive and enthusiastic about themselves and fellow team members. This is not attributed to having undergone some strange therapy. Rather, these feelings stem from the fact that they are now coordinating their efforts more successfully, and as a result, see direct effects on their ability to meet patient needs directly or through their efforts as a support group to deliverers.

The Managerial Role in Team Development

The management group (e.g. clinic director, medical director, administrator, etc.) of a health care organization in which teams are used plays a critical role in the total process of team development at two specific points, at the time of getting started and at that point when the after effects must be dealt with.

Getting Started : Top Management Commitment

Health administrators and managers are under severe environmental constraints which represent major obstacles to freeing up the time required for team development. Management's response to these constraints confronts directly the issue of its commitment to interdisciplinary care. Some managers argue that team development is important but teams should do it on their own time — lunch hours, evenings, week- ends. The subtle (but powerful) message thereby communicated is that management is not committed to finding ways to support a program that the team perceives as high priority. The team is likely to lose some of its own commitment in such a situation. On the other hand, managerial commitment to freeing up the time required, sets in motion a positive, self-reinforcing motivational pattern for the teams who will be engaged in the team development program.

Some After Effects : Managing Developed Teams

The act of offering and implementing a team development program represents an organizational, as well as a team, intervention. A particular team is only a sub-system within a larger organizational system. 9 Developed teams are very likely to want to use their newfound strength to improve the organization of which they are a part.

In effect, what happened in some of the field test cases reported here was that teams began to question the rationale and usefulness of certain policies, decisions, and procedures. Once developed, the teams felt capable of handling more responsibil- ity and sought ways to be more autonomous and self-sufficient. It is important to point out, however, that while team members expressed these feelings, they also noted that such action was not directed towards "taking over the organization" or "doing the administrating ourselves." The intent in these instances was to make organiza- tional goals and administrative functions more effective and relevant to the team's specific setting, patient population, and mixture of disciplines. Nevertheless, several administrators, quite appropriately, reacted to these phenomena with initial hesitancy and concern. They felt as though teams were "ganging up on them," and de- grading the role of administration. While initial tensions existed in several set- tings, these tensions did not necessarily lead to negative results. In five of the organizations where teams completed the program, administrators either initiated changes in organization structure and policy to facilitate team and administrative functioning or sought their own training programs as a result of viewing changes in their team's functioning.

Conclusion

The results described of a team development program are based on field tests with thirteen teams. These results support the belief that "developed" health teams are more efficient and effective deliverers of care than non-developed teams. The cost of this development in terms of time is not insignificant and must be weighed against the potential returns. The contention is that to be effective, health care teams (and, for that matter, any team) must spend some time in planned developmental activities. All teams spend much of their time and energy coping with the problems of interdependence — developmental programs can help them do it better.

TABLE ONE
DEMOGRAPHIC CHARACTERISTICS OF TEST SITES (N=13)

	TYPE OF SETTING	LOCATION	SIZE	COMPOSITION*
1.	Community health centerde livery team	Massachuset ts	10	I. Pe , NP, PeNP . PsNp , FHW ,
				SW, HE. TC
2.	Community health cener delivery team	Massachuset ts	10	I . Pe, NP , PeNP. PsKP, FHW ,
				SW. NE, TC
3.	Community health center delivery team	Massachuset ts	10	Pe. RN. LPN, NP. NA, FHW,
				SW, MHW
4.	Community health center delivery team	Florida	6	I, Pe. RN, FHW, SW
S.	Community health center delivery team	New York City	14	T, Pe . D, N, FHW. CHA. S
6.	Community health center delivery team	New York City	14	I, Pe . 0, N. FHW, CHA. S
7.	Community health center delivery team	Manitoba, Canada	8	I, NP, PHN. SW , HE
8.	Comprehensive mental health center delivery team (day shift)	Virginia	13	RN, LPN , MHT, MHA (psychiatrists serve as consultants)
9.	Comprehensive mental health center delivery team (evening shift)	Virginia	6	RN, LPN, MHT, MHA (psychiatrists serve a s consultants)
10.	Comprehensive mental health center delivery team (night shift)	Virginia	4	RN, LPN. ~IT. MHA (psychiatrists serve as consultants)
11.	University-based clinic delivery team	Indiana	12	1. RN. NP. S
12. 13.	Teaching/delivery team in a university setting Administrative team of a prepared group practice (CHMO)	Nevada Missouri	9 3	1, N. Ps, SW. HE, MT Medical Director, Program Direc tor, Business Administrator

COMPOSITION KEY TO TABLE ONE

1.	D = Dentist	11.	NP = Nurse Practitioner
2.	FHW = Family/Community Health Worker	12.	Pe = Pediatrician
3.	HE = Health Educator	13.	PeNP = Pediatric Nurse Practitioner
4.	I = Internist	14.	PHN = Public Health Nurse
5.	LPN = Licensed Practical Nurse	15.	Ps = Psychologist
6.	MEA = Mental Health Aide Practitioner	16.	PSNP = Psychiatric Nurse
7.	MHT = Mental Health Technician	17.	RN = Registered Nurse
8.	MHW = Mental Health Worker I	18.	S = Secretary/Receptionist
9.	MT = Medical Technician	19.	SW = Social Worker
10.	NA = Nursing Assistant	20.	Tc = Team Coordinator

FOOTNOTES

1. J.J. Horwitz, Team Practice and the Specialist (Springfield, Illinois: C.C. Thomas Publishers, 1970).
2. B. Siegel, "Organization of the Primary Care Team," Pediatric Clin . , May, 1974.
3. H. Wise, "The Primary Care Health Team," Arch, of Int. Med ., Vol. 130, September, 1972, pp. 438-444.
4. A.W. Parker, The Team Approach to Primary Health Care (monograph) (University Extension, University of California, 1972).
5. I. Rubin, M. Plovnick, R. Fry, Improving the Coordination of Care: A Program for Health Team Development (Cambridge, MA: Ballinger Publishing Co., Spring, 1975).
6. R. Beckhard, D. Lake, "Short and Long-Range Effects of a Team Development Effort," in Social Intervention , ed. by H. Hornstein et. al. (New York: Free Press, 1971).
7. S. Seashore, "Group Cohesiveness as a Factor in Industrial Morale and Productivity," in Readings in Organizational and Industrial Psychology , by G. Yukl and K. Weping (New York: Oxford University Press, 1971).
8. F. Friedlander, "The Impact of Organizational Training Laboratories Upon the Effectiveness and Interaction of Ongoing Work Group," Personnel Psych ., Vol. 20, No. 3, 1967.
9. R. Blake et. al., Managing Intergroup Conflict in Industry (Houston, Texas: Gulf- Publishing, 1964).

10. R. Fry, B. Lech, "An Organizational Development Approach to Improving the Effectiveness of Neighborhood Health Care Teams: A Pilot Program," Unpublished Master's Thesis, M.I.T. , 1971.

11. H. Wise et. al., Making Health Teams Work (Cambridge, MA:Ballinger Publishing Co., 1974).

12. S.P. Simson et. al., "The Development of a Primary Health Care Team," Prim. Care, Vol. 1, No. 3, September, 1974.

13 M. Tichy, Health Care Teams: An Annotated Bibliography (New York: Praeger Publishers, 1974).

14. I. Rubin, R. Beckhard, "Factors Influencing the Effectiveness of Health Teams, Milbank Mem. Fund Quarterly , Vol. 1, No. 3, July, 1972, pp. 287-316.

15. H. Wise et. al., op. cit., Chapter Two, pp. 27-61.

16. J. Forward, A. Zander, "Choice of Unattainable Group Goals and Effects on Performance," Org. Behavior & Human Performance , Vol. 6, 1971, pp. 184-199.

17. A. Zander, Motives and Goals in Groups (New York: Academic Press, 1971).

18. R. Mager, Goal Analysis (Belmont, California: Fearon, 1972).

19. Kahn et. al., Organizational Stress: Studies in Role Conflict and Ambiguity (New York: Wiley Press, 1964).

20. N.R.F. Maier, Problem Solving and Creativity Individuals and Groups (Belmont, California: Brooks/Cole, 1970).

21. B.E. Collins, H. Guetzkow, A Social Psychology of Group Process for Decision Making (New York: John Wiley and Sons, Inc., 1964).

22. F.E. Fiedler, Theory of Leadership Effectiveness (New York: McGraw Hill, Inc., 1967).

23. W.R. Bion, Experiences in Groups (New York: Basic Books, Inc., 1959).

24. W.C. Schutz, "Interpersonal Underworld," Harvard Business Review, Vol. 36, No. 4, July-August, 1958, pp. 123-135.

25. H. Wise et. al., op. it.

26. R. Beckhard, Organization Development: Strategies and Models (Reading, MA: Addison-Wesley Publishing Co., 1969).
27. I. Rubin, M. Plovnick, R. Fry, "Initiating Planned Change in Health Care Systems," Journal of Applied Behavioral Science , Vol. 10, No. 1, 1974.
28. N.S. Stearns, "Educational Consultation: A Team Approach to Stimulating Hospital Medical Staff Involvement in Health Care Problems of the Poor," Med. Care , Vol. 10, No. 2, March-April, 1972, pp. 179-185.
29. R. Beckhard, "Organizational Issues in the Team Delivery of Comprehensive Health Care," Milbank Mem. Fund Quarterly , Vol. 1, No. 3, Part 1, July, 1972.